HOPEZINE

A LITTLE BOOK OF HOPE

Curated by Erica Crompton

CONTENTS

Chapter One: Hope For Suicidal Thoughts 9

Chapter 2: Hope With Mental Illness 33

Chapter Three: Hope For All Disabilities 65

Chapter Four: Hope With A Criminal Record 89

INTRODUCTION

Hopezine is a small, printed independent magazine and blog by me, Erica Crompton, a journalist with schizoaffective disorder who survived a suicide attempt. This book is a small selection of the best stories, poems and vignettes published in my magazine and on my blog at Hopezine.com.

Launched at an NHS suicide prevention conference in November 2018 at the Bet365 stadium in Staffordshire (UK), Hopezine aims to share stories from people who have survived adversity in all its forms to offer hope for all people with mental illnesses or disabilities.

It was in that previous summer 2018 I heard of the sad passing of two friends from my childhood to suicide. I'd stayed in touch with both occasionally through Facebook. I do a lot of mental health campaigning, which I post on social media, as I myself have attempted suicide. After hearing the sad news that summer, it felt like I wasn't doing enough. I felt a burning desire to help a community feeling low to feel better. I decided, as a mental health campaigner, that I'd use my own experience surviving a suicide attempt to try to help others understand myself and survivors better.

So, I started to write and give talks about suicide – what works and what doesn't; what helped me during my suicide attempt, what didn't help; and how I came to feel so low in the first place. Today I continue to write about surviving suicide for most quality newspapers including The Guardian, The Mail on Sunday, The Los Angeles Times and The New York Times.

My 'Hopezine' is trying to reach out to people on my social media and in my community and beyond to offer advice and uplifting reads. I wished to collect some stories of hope from people who had failed suicide attempts and show how they're still here and still smiling. I hoped to show that you're never alone in the dark – indeed if you look closely, you'll find myself and others here. There's always hope for a brighter future. It doesn't matter who you are, what you do or where you've been – hope is universal, and we all see the same sunshine no matter who we are.

I was especially pleased with the cover artwork for the inaugural issue of Hopezine by the amazing artist Pure Evil who donated his neon pink 'Mr Messy' to the issue for free. The Mr Messy, rendered in spray paint, felt fitting and I thought that we can all feel like Mr Messy at times. The trick is, I gestured in the issue's Editor's letter, like our cover model, to just keep on smiling.

Today, from my little bungalow in Staffordshire, I'm delighted that Hopezine continues to grow with sponsorship from Fintel, a finance company that helps businesses. Fintel's CEO is Matthew Timmins, a friend from school who had also heard of our friends' passings to suicide in that grim summer of 2018. With Matt's help I'm now sixteen issues in, with many different themes from spirituality to the USA and online dating to help guide, advise and give readers a boost.

I've proudly managed to pay cash to artists and writers with mental health concerns in the UK and beyond. In the spiritual issue, for winter 2020, I published cover art by Bristol artist George J Harding and asked readers to try to decode the hidden messages in his work. I've focused on what can be done by turning on, tuning in and copping out. I gathered a cohort of Hare Krishna devotees from the Krishna Eco Farm in Scotland to examine spiritual lives without material trappings. I wrote my own meditations on how lockdown has made hermits of all of us.

Since we started, we've received press coverage for our work in The Daily Mail, Happiful Magazine, Scotland's Daily Record, and the Lancet Psychiatry. We've worked with academics to promote citizen science and student photographers at Stafford College to promote hope for young people.

Since 2018, we've grown from a team of one to a team of two with a wide variety of expert and lived experience contributors. In September 2021, wheelchair-user Paul Nicholls got onboard as Accessibility Consultant, and we launched an accessible travel element to Hopezine on a trip to Belfast, marked with a special print edition dedicated to the city seen in a wheelchair.

This book highlights the best, most hopeful stories and vignettes from Hopezine in four chapters of different survivor and marginalised voices – hope for those with... suicidal thoughts, with mental illness, with disabilities and with criminal records. Whatever your struggle, you can learn hard-won lessons of hope and survival from those who lived to tell the tale within these pages.

So put the kettle on, sit back and let us uplift you!

Erica x

CHAPTER ONE

HOPE FOR SUICIDAL THOUGHTS

Hope when all hope is lost

By GC

In early June 2019, I came home from hospital without the twins I was expecting. My beautiful son and daughter were born alive, but too small to survive for long.

I can't find adequate words or phrases - in this language at least - to describe how dark and devastating that sort of bereavement is. While recovering in the immediate aftermath, we were constantly encouraged to have 'hope'. But what is hope? I kept hearing that word so often that it became an abstract, nonsense word. And then it irked me.

Looking back over the past year, there are ways to let the light in when the dark suffocates you. You might find them inside yourself, or externally. Hope is rooted in optimism - and when that evaporates, as it did - grit. Although I'm a naturally optimistic person, it's really not as if I thought there was better around the corner; I felt not so much like dying, but not being here to exist either. No before, present or after. All I could feel was a sense of moving through time.

Just know that if there's an imperative within you to keep moving through a dark time, there's no obligation to do it quickly and certainly not at a speed convenient to other people. Hope is hidden in self-soothing when the pain becomes too much. It was there after an intense rainstorm... a rainbow, or twin rainbows, reflections of each other, would appear and loom large in the sky. In those moments, I smile. Rainbows can only happen after moving through a turbulent time. That's why they're a symbol of 2020 - and also a symbol of new life after loss.

My start to motherhood was the worst it could possibly be, and even now I fend off clumsy attempts to ease my pain or get me to look past it. You see your pain the way you want and need to and handle it on your terms. Never compromise on that.

My son, born almost a year to the day his siblings were, looks a lot like them, which delights me and breaks my heart in equal measure. I write this after another night of disrupted sleep, which is absolutely normal for me - but so is seeing my baby smile when he wakes up and I say, 'Good morning!' Some days, I can float along on a feeling of optimism, and I can project that onto my child. I was fortunate enough to be able to bring another new life into this world, which is certainly a bleak place in 2020. And other days, when I'm moving through the weight of sadness and it feels like all hope is lost, an imperative remains.

You don't have to 'move on', but sometimes moving is all you can do, whether it's forwards, sideways, diagonally. Sometimes it might even be a bit backwards. Tune into that imperative and pay attention to it. Grab on to it with all your might.

It's a wonderful life

By Graham Morgan

Every day, when I am alone, I speak into the silence and say, "I want to die" and every day that I am beside the tracks at Central Station, I think; 'You are disgusting' and I think of throwing myself in front of the train that will take me home.

And I am meant to say something about this that might give comfort? Maybe I can, I do not know. My CPN often says it would be good for me to talk to a psychologist, to deal with my negativity and, when she speaks to her, the psychologist says my delusions are so entrenched, that talking about them just makes it more real and painful, and I tend to agree.

What keeps me alive? Well, for me, it is taking medication that I do not willingly take but which I know keeps me from a reality I would do anything to avoid. But far more than that is the everyday so many of us do not have. For me it is Wendy, my partner, giving me a kiss when I give her a coffee in the morning. It is Dash, my dog, leaping up for our cuddle when we say hello after my night in the snoring room. It is also the hub bub and the drama of getting the children ready for school.

When I left my wife, I was nearing fifty and was tired and lonely and traumatized: when I lost contact with my son, it was the worst thing that had ever happened to me. In those years and when I was in hospital; when I knew that I would never ever be in a relationship again; knew I would always be lonely; that I would grow old and frail and lose the few friends I had. I did not look forward to my life. My world was mechanical, lifeless. And yet, somehow, despite my sadness and with the help of new friends and the help of my new CPN, my life gained some colour.

I dared the dream of reaching out for friendship. I learned the basics of mortgages and buying clothes and books in charity shops; of finding wonder that I could go to bed at two in the morning without comment and that I could eat a pizza so laden with cheese it dripped onto the plate. I learnt to do the things that pleased and delighted me. I walked long walks along the beach. I sat on the bench at the peat rich curve of the river Nairn. I sat silent but welcome with the parents and the dogs and the children at the Links café on a weekend. And I met Wendy - and I realized that love was possible for me and, to my astonishment that someone could love me, could want me, could enjoy texting me till two in the morning, could promise the first thing we would do would be to kiss when she got off the train to see me in Inverness.

And this may not be for you; it may never happen. It may not be your solution and it certainly is not my cure but, when life is beyond grey, when you cannot and do not want hope there may, one day, be things that give light to your day. Whether that be the feel of frost on your face on a winter's day, a walk with the dog, a book you finally have the energy to read, the extravagance of chips and curry sauce, a friend who gives you a hug or a stranger in the street who gives you the first smile in months, it is possible.

When I was at my worst, I had no idea of the impact my death would cause other people. It was meaningless, until a few years ago when my brother shouted down the phone at me when I said I wanted to stop my medication. He shouted and almost cried when he asked, 'Did I not know that the whole family waited for the call that said I was dead when I was in hospital again?' And I never knew. I never knew that anyone would have cared, would have been hurt by my death and so, when I wait for the train to come by, I pause, I think of my partner who I never thought I would have waiting for me to get home from work. I think to myself 'This is wonderful!' I hope so much that you can have this one day too.

A failure at suicide counts as success at life!

By Alan Hartley

At the end of my school days, I left after failing all my A Levels. However, I did get a job and, indeed, had several good jobs, but none of them lasted because of my incompetence and I went from one job to another before finally losing my job and, as a result, my house. At about the same time, I also fell out with my girlfriend.

This put me in a downward spiral and there were several suicide attempts with several short stays in a psychiatric hospital over a period of years, but the most memorable involved taking tablets. I took a lot but then I sat outside in the garden at home whilst waiting for the tablets to take effect. While sitting there, in the sun, I was in turmoil with thoughts of what would happen if I failed and survived.

This was about 35 years ago and, admittedly, I have been on medication for Paranoid Schizophrenia ever since, but I have since had some good jobs and worked as an Aquatics Centre Manager, a sales representative, a website builder and a self-published author. Now, somewhat older and in retirement, I am doing voluntary work at a rural centre for Adults with Learning Disabilities and writing for a local talking newspaper. I have many friends of all sorts around me, enjoy playing competitive darts, looking after my allotment and, as they say, I am comfortable in my retirement with a reasonably sized private pension fund to supplement my income. I am living in a lovely bungalow that I own and driving a nice little car that is all mine. LIFE is GOOD!

A true story

By a loving friend and writer

Let's call her Jane. She was, in her teens, shy and extremely sensitive. She hated the way she looked, couldn't look at herself in the mirror as she thought she was fat and ugly. These thoughts led to anorexia, a serious eating disorder where people can starve themselves. Jane's situation got to the point where she could barely stand up, let alone go out.

All this made her problems worse, leading to depression with suicidal thoughts. At a low point, Jane attempted to take her life. She was then hospitalised with girls who had similar problems. Unfortunately, even in hospital, the trauma continued. She had a drip but still found ways to regurgitate. Jane loathed herself and couldn't stop crying out: 'Why won't anyone understand!'

Finally, however, she had reached a weight that wasn't life threatening and she started to see things in a different light, although the feeling of loathing never left. For a long time, Jane still wasn't eating and she was still restricting her daily calories, always restricting herself to the bare minimum! Jane wasn't confident and was still suffering with depression, anxiety and other problems relating to how she saw herself.

But the story doesn't end there. Eventually, our heroine got a job where she was meeting the public and having to interact with people – this made her begin to feel more confident. She made some good friends who helped her to talk more about how she felt on her dark days. The new job and friends helped Jane to feel better about herself as these friends didn't judge her. Instead, they accepted her and supported her. Their love was unconditional. Jane got better and better.

Isn't it good to hear that Jane is now a model for clothes, is married with children of her own? Jane's friend who tells us this touching story says: 'Such is life: when things seem as dark as they can be, don't give up because you never know what's waiting for you further down the road.'

A musical note

By Corin Liall Douieb AKA The Last Skeptik

Making and listening to music has helped me in so many different ways during my life. From the big sledgehammer traumas to the underlying buzz of anxiety that I sometimes struggle to successfully manage. Ever since I was little, music has been the granter of permissions for me to feel emotions.

Sometimes I struggle in a quiet room to cry or be in my own skin, or process pain, but music (in any form, including film soundtracks) somehow makes the guilt of feeling depressed go away and transports me into a hyper-real land where I'm allowed to let it all out.

When I first had trouble and had to leave school aged 14, I channelled everything into my simmering love for the power songs had over me, and fully followed my passion for writing. That intense loneliness and sadness I felt, the self-harm I endured both physically and mentally, it was lessened and de-knotted by writing lyrics and music. Still today, I'll go for weeks where I struggle to make anything at all because I'm not quite ready to face the truth head on.

I recently finished writing my new album entirely inspired by the grief experience after a breakup, and, in exactly the same way it helped me at 14, it has done the same now. I almost don't have a choice but to write it down. Whilst not in the same suicidal state that maybe I had been in my younger years, I was at my wits end with my health anxiety. My spiral thinking and panic attacks were at their worst.

Listening to the songs I had made were a stronger version of me telling me at my lowest ebb that I could do this. That these things have happened before, and they will happen again, and I've always survived. Sometimes teaching yourself to self-soothe is the most powerful tool you can give yourself. By no means am I a master at this - and even as I write this, waiting for the album to be released, I am yet again at arm's length with my creativity, high in anxiety and not able to face the mirror that is music. It's in these moments that I reach for the emergency playlists I make, something to guide me to until I'm stronger. Through the years I have sometimes forgotten the reason why I create and get bogged down with sales or promoting or not getting the success I dreamt of, then I try and remind myself that creation is the most helpful therapy I've ever had, and that even if no one likes anything I make, it has already served its purpose. And I've already won.

Why I take my medication every day

By Erica Crompton

I've made the artwork opposite to show how my brain might look when I'm unwell with psychosis. I call these collages the 'brain surgery series' as, to make them, I take a scalpel to pictures of people in magazines! Since 1999, I've taken different measures of antipsychotic medication to treat psychosis or the brain explosions you see in my artwork and this means that, today, I'm able to live my life without too many symptoms of my illness.

For me, I don't worry too much about side effects as they've always been outweighed by the benefits of taking pills: being able to get out and about, being able to take part in paid work, being independent and, best of all, keeping on top of my relationships with loved ones. A prescription and a therapeutic relationship with my psychiatrist also mean I can access employment support benefits as stress can cause a relapse so I am advised not to work too hard! My psychiatrist has told me I'll be on medication for life but that there's still hope to reduce my dosage if things improve. I hope one day that happens but I'm in no hurry! Working with psychologists and a psychiatrist has been one of my best decisions in life as, on the whole, I consider myself in a much happier place than when my psychosis was left untreated.

My sunshine

By Erica Crompton

It was a ray of light through the curtains. I'd drank a poisonous concoction just minutes before I glimpsed the spring sun, powerfully penetrating the kitsch pink daisy printed curtains in my large bedroom in a flat share in a rundown part of Birmingham. That light spoke to me when no words could describe the state I'd been in over the last two weeks – funny then that it was also the wordless sun that communicated so much hope to me on that day.

In a flash, I'd called an ambulance. I saw in that sunlight my youth. I was 29 years old and I'd seen my situation in an altogether different light after the rain and clouds of the last few weeks had lifted at some incredibly fortuitous timing. When I tell people about that moment, they think the psychosis may have lifted but it hadn't. For the following weeks, I believed any written words I read – including articles about Lady Gaga in The Daily Mirror, a newspaper I had previously contributed too – were written in an abstract way to hurt me. But the sunlight, at the moment in time when I needed it the most, warmed my cheeks and melted away some of the psychosis and all the self-loathing that brings for just long enough time for me to call 999.

In psychiatry, they call the ups and downs of 'paranoid schizophrenia', what I was later diagnosed with, as 'the course of the illness'. I call it 'the snakes and ladders of life'. Sure, I am up and down perhaps more than most.

However, at the end of the day when the sun is setting, I'm so glad for something as simple as a ray of spring sunlight during a crisis I had one day ten years ago. It saved my life and, in hindsight, I'm so glad it did for there's love, friendship and always others to help. After the dawn of a failed suicide, there is sunshine.

Never say never

By Erica Crompton

Having just been diagnosed with a severe mental illness and struggling to hold down a day job, I sought escapism watching Spooks. It's a TV programme I'd downloaded for after working each day in an office in southeast London where I also lived. The days were hard and I enjoyed Spooks so much I found myself falling for one of the lead characters who, a quick Google search later, told me was played by the actor Rupert Penry Jones. The catch was that my evening escapism was just that.

The more I watched the more my heart started to ache, for I would never meet Rupert in real life – he was always behind my TV screen. As the days passed, I'd soon watched every episode but still dreamt of Rupert and knew I'd never meet him. I just had to get on with my life.

As you'll know, London property is expensive so, not long after I'd watched all the Spooks episodes, I took on a weekend job as an usher at The Unicorn Theatre- a delightful, brand-new space where children can learn through plays. Within two weeks of getting the job and doing my training, the opening night arrived. I couldn't believe it – there were loads of celebrities including Cherie and Tony Blair. As I watched the cameras flash at the incoming celebrities, I noticed a family of three walking towards the scene and recognised the father. It was Rupert! He was coming to the opening night as he himself had a young child interested to see plays. I was terribly star-struck! But just in awe.

As everyone took their seats for the first ever play, I took my position outside ready to sell ice-creams - and then Rupert popped out and asked me where the gentleman's bathroom was. I will never forget this evening and my thoughts about Rupert previously so, when I'm having a bad day or thinking this or that is impossible, I remind myself of meeting Rupert. Never say never.

Helping others is helping myself

By Nutan Modha

It's taken a while to finally put fingers to keyboard as I do find it painful to look back. Some on the outside looking in can adopt a variety of opinions on our characters. The newspapers seem to see fit in blowing cases involving the mentally ill like me out of proportion. It is mine and our wish that 'Hopezine' gives those papers a run for their money!

The current climate of lone agents brandishing knives on subways and on our streets are seemingly the stuff of terror inducing headlines. With a lack of motivation, bouts of the blues and possibly no work in our future lives, I have found that healing takes time. Much of it involves being proactive, even when you would rather not. Ruminating and back peddling occurs. The illness that takes over your mind and becomes a fear rather than the calling, a calling which has been shredded. This wipe-out may as well dishonour the human.

We become full of emotion, so much so that we splinter. It's a time to be brave and, if recurrent journal keeping is helpful, I'll give it a go. Never on a PC but in a lovely book. I have kept a diary since I was first unwell in 1993. It's helpful and a nice way to pass time looking through the years.

Getting back on my feet after several suicide attempts has involved helping others at the same time. Starting a group in London for mental health support and also getting work after volunteering. The field of mental health seems to be on the tip of everyone's tongue these days, with papers talking about long and impossible waiting lists.

In my opinion, if you stand high enough, you can see a legion of us who have survived and are more than willing to lend a hand. As Ron Coleman quoted 'We're experts by experience'. Of that, I'm certain. I'm also certain that I'm never alone these days – we all suffer and we should all help one another.

Stories of hope from Harplands Hospital, Staffordshire

Messages of hope from patients who have been there too

- This too shall pass.
- Talk to your spouse or a friend, you can't do this alone – don't do it!
- Depression is like a thick fog around you. Sometimes all you can do is have patience – wait for the fog to lift so you can get your bearings again and put your life back on track.
- Know you are someone's child or friend and think of the pain you'll leave behind.
- Try to focus your anger on something you are good at.
- If your problems are debt related, get help with bills with CAB or Starfish.

- Try to eat well and know there is hope no matter what your faith.

- For family and friends, you can get help from the Carer's Hub.

- With OCD, it takes many forms such as intrusive thoughts, obsessive washing, feeling someone is watching you, fear of germs and dirt. If you're feeling like this, seek help as soon as possible. You will be prescribed drugs and possibly therapy – there is help out there, so please find it.

- You are unique. You are special and loved. We believe in you.

- It's OK to feel not okay – recovery is possible and achievable.

- Don't give up as you don't know what's round the corner.

- Don't bottle it up. You won't be a burden – share your pain and lighten the load on your shoulders.

Identity Lost

By Jim Leftwich

Clasping at air
All thought in celestial space
My thoughts I do not own
All originality is banal
It makes no difference
Locked inside or put upon the page
Puncturing the rind of the mind
Thoughts flow in
But others are sucked out - I stand alone
Solidarity is a paltry promise
The devils of the mind command isolation
The neon emotions of dysfunction I hold and abate but it does not dull the suffering
The diaspora of feigning a sound mind
Has led me full circle
The tribe I abandoned will perhaps take me back
Finally, I am posed to pull the switch
The one that governs dread and anticipation
Can lead to balance of peace of mind
The quest for openness
The desire for the porous borders of free thought
Smile on my progress and ensure the fight continues

Storms make people stronger

By James Leftwich, CEO NoLongerLonely.com

I've never tried kill myself. However, I certainly have thought about it. I'm not a religious person but I do have a belief that life is quite precious and that abandoning it is something of a violation. Suicidality is a repudiation of long-term thinking. Someone on the brink cannot see beyond their immediate circumstance. It's a cliche to talk about positive thinking in such circumstances and a recommendation that a suicidal person would find almost comical. However, the real key to overcoming a severe mental health crisis is to accept long-term thinking and undergo a planning process with an understanding that success is incremental and won't happen overnight.

I was hospitalised one time when I was 22 years old. I quickly found myself ostracised by friends and even family. As I came over to the realisation that this mental illness would not abate and may even worsen over time, I made a crucial decision that I would not succumb to it. No matter how much I struggled, I maintained a goal (fantasy?) that I would emerge the victor. At the time, I likened it to the hero of the Count of Monte Cristo, who suffers but triumphs in the end over his doubters. Despite many hiccups along the way I've never lost sight of the ultimate goal. It has required patience and a willingness to endure very uncomfortable circumstances. In hindsight, I see a very logical procession.

Growing up, I did quite well in school. I could always count on my intellectual ability. It enabled me to finish my bachelor's degree after leaving the hospital. Many doubted my ability to do that. Showing that people were wrong to doubt my abilities became a motivating factor. Despite getting my diploma, I felt quite low. I still compared myself to childhood friends who were becoming doctors, lawyers and successful businessmen. At the time, I could barely manage a cashier job at a hardware store.

Reminding myself about incremental success, I brainstormed a situation that would entail fairly low stress and would take advantage of my cerebral nature. I settled upon a bookstore. This was a superb decision. I still had health benefits and housing subsidies so money was not a worry. It became a place I looked forward to going to and allowed me to re-acclimate to social situations. It built confidence.

After two years there, I became restless. I still had an overall urge to prove my doubters wrong and regain my status among old friends. I tried to figure out the next step I could take that would allow me take advantage of my natural talents, was still fairly low stress, would pay better and what could amount to a real career. I settled on librarianship.

I set about methodically earning credits and, before I knew it, I had a master's degree. I found a profession that profoundly interested me. Schoolwork itself was not very stressful but work environments during my internship triggered my paranoia and urge to socially withdraw. I realized I would have to approach the workplace delicately. I was surprised to learn my local public library was hiring part-time librarians. I set about working 15 hours a week at the reference desk. I began to slowly learn the ways of libraries. At the same time, I found it easier to look people in the eye and not let my symptoms overwhelm my social encounters.

A chance encounter led me to working at a small local college library. After three years of part-time work, I became a full-time employee and shed all my public benefits. I had made it. I was a full tax-paying American citizen. Soon after, I became Director of that library. While in hindsight, that was perhaps too vast a leap to make as much of the responsibility triggered my symptoms, it appears the same on my resume. I stayed there 10 years.

My hopeful message boils down to three things: have a long-term plan that you methodically go about implementing; be willing to put yourself into uncomfortable situations; celebrate small successes even if you only you realize their import; use naysayers as motivation to exceed expectations; don't trust clinical appraisals of how dire your circumstances might be; acknowledge and accept that you are facing more impediments to success than most people.

CHAPTER 2

HOPE WITH MENTAL ILLNESS

The nook

By Erica Crompton

We knew as soon as we heard Ms Swain had booked in for a house viewing that destiny was at play. My lovely home and safe space, a wee white cottage in a leafy street was up for sale and, if I'd had any doubts about selling-up and moving somewhere more accessible with Paul, the arrival of Ms Swain on the viewing scene put them all to rest.

That's because the name 'Swain' holds significance for Paul and me – ever since I danced like "a swan" on Paul's 40th birthday, just a few months after we made our relationship official on Facebook. We would laugh and recall this when we saw the name 'swan' on a pub facade or a swan swimming elegantly on a lake. Soon after, I spotted Swan Street on a drive to the West Midlands safari park and got excited to bring the memory of the swan dance back again – a little too excited: "Swain Street! Swain Street!" I blurted, and of course we fell about laughing at my mispronunciation.

We'd later watch Jonathan Swain present the news on our TV or see the name Swain on a shop front as we drove past or even shout the name 'Swain' as we drove past those swans in the countryside near where Paul lived at the time. 'Swain' had established itself in our love language that only we knew.

My cottage had already been on the market for a few months; one sale had fallen through at the last minute which had been so stressful. We were worried we'd lose the accessible bungalow I'd put a deposit on – the only one I could afford. Like I said at the start, we knew destiny was at play as soon as we heard about Ms Swain taking an interest in the cottage. We couldn't know for sure, but it seemed so promising and such a remarkable coincidence. Ms Swain did go ahead and buy the cottage; I hear she's settled and loves it which feels meaningful to me. Paul and I went on to move into our bungalow which we love, too. Sometimes our destiny is divine by design.

The bevelled-edge mirror

By Erica Crompton

Ever since I was a child, I've had an appreciation of antiques. I grew up with parents who loved car boot sales, charity shops and all things vintage (before it became cool). More recently, I'd bought myself a tiny, white cottage in a little village in Staffordshire, to be closer to my family. Here, I decided to continue the family tradition of vintage interiors and antiques. I decided that the statement mirrors in the house should all be bevelled-edged mirrors from the 1930s. These mirrors are usually heavy, wood-backed and frameless with cut-glass shaping around the edge and a chunky steel chain to hang them on that you can also see when the mirrors are hung.

The first 1930s mirrors I got were expensive second-hand ones from eBay – around £45 each and I bought two – one for the lounge and one for the bathroom. I still needed one for the master bedroom. It wasn't long before I felt it pressing to furnish the bedroom with a mirror as I had a guest who was visiting - I no longer had time to wait for the post from eBay. So, I went into town to see. if by chance, I could find a vintage mirror in the charity shop. I looked in all of them, and there are a lot of second-hand shops in the nearby town. I hardly saw any mirrors at all. In the end I was thinking about spending £100 for one in Laura Ashley but it wasn't a patch on my small collection of bevelled-edged mirrors.

Before I went to buy the expensive one, I thought I'd give one last charity shop a go – Dougie Mac. As soon as I walked in a song I love was playing (Castles in the Sky by Ian Van Dahl) and I suddenly felt I might find what I'm looking for. I instinctively went to the back of the shop and moved a big, framed picture out the way. And there it was! My bevelled-edged mirror, a nice big one for the master bedroom – just £10! It felt amazing finding such a bargain at just the right time. However, shortly afterwards, my cat knocked the bathroom mirror off the wall and it smashed. I'm kinda superstitious and wondered if I'd get bad luck but remembered how fortuitous it was to find my bargain mirror for the master room and thought twice before worrying about my luck. I decided to return to Dougie Mac again, in case they had another nice mirror.

And now I really do know I'm lucky – I found another bevelled edge mirror in there as soon as I walked in... for £3.10! I got it immediately and hung it in the bathroom as soon as I got home. I've come to see why my family love antiques and charity shops so much. It's not just about having nice things – it's the thrill and feeling of being lucky involved in hunting for a bargain and finding one.

Finding hope with mantras

By Katrina Robinson

I can honestly say fear no longer frightens me the way it did that day many years ago when I realised I had apparently inherited my mother and her family's tendency to mood disorders.

When you are young and inexperienced you think that having any mental illness guarantees a terrible life. Now I'm much further along in my mental health journey, I've learnt that was the fear speaking, not reality. I want to encourage anyone feeling that fear.

What has helped? More than one thing. The right medication, a supportive husband, a gentle work discipline, keeping active, my own wish to recover.

Plus, simple but true mantras:

- Depression is a self-limiting illness. It will go.

- I've been through this before. I can do it again.

- Bad feelings change. They disappear and go. If you can hold onto the fact that you feel a tiny bit better at this moment than you did lying awake at 4am this morning then a crucial life-skill is within your grasp.

With anxiety and panic attacks I've learnt not to battle them as this only adds to the tension. Instead, I distract myself by doing some little tasks that keep my mind and hands occupied, like sorting out the cutlery drawer which was an idea from a sympathetic GP. The worst of the feelings will have begun to evaporate by the end.

Mantras range from the mundane to the sublime. People talk about faith as though it were a sort of simplistic spiritual splint but actually, I find it shows life is nuanced and full of mysterious depths. Anyone with a faith who has suffered has asked, 'Why does God let me suffer like this?' The only possible answer has to be, 'How should I know? Job asked the same question thousands of years ago.'

I recently discovered some mantra-like prayers from the writer Elizabeth Goudge, herself a mental health sufferer and survivor.

Here's how I think they can help whether you interpret them in a religious way, or more as a response to the mystery of life:

'God — Love — is a trinity, so here are three prayers of three words each. Short and easy to remember:

Lord, have mercy :	=	Asking for help and being aware it may not come in a form you expect.
Thee I adore :	=	Recognising that to be alive is ultimately a privilege.
Into thy hands :	=	Practising a radical acceptance.

During dark times, if you can hold onto these words in a way that makes sense to you, something changes for the better.

And if ever I feel I am stumbling along a dark, dark tunnel, I remember the prisoner in The Shawshank Redemption who eventually tunnelled his way through what seemed an impossible distance.

His explanation: 'Time and persistence. That's all it takes.'

@Part2LoveLife

www.katrinarobinson.co.uk/P2YL

Sparkly poem

By Knuckles

Everyone has a spark inside
A spiritual guiding light
To illuminate the paths ahead
On our darkest nights
It doesn't matter if you pray
Or don't believe in God at all
Awakening to your inner light
Is like answering a helping call.

Come fly with me

By Erica Crompton

Some years ago, I attempted to board a flight to Ibiza but had to check out at the last minute due to some mild hallucinations (thinking I could see people from the past). I'll admit, it wasn't very well planned on my part – the flight from Manchester airport was on a Friday night and of all the places to visit I'd chosen the party island… well, I hate crowds and rowdy hen parties!

It's actually not uncommon to fall ill sans flight – there's been a paper in Psychiatric Times recently that looks into the subject of travelling with a severe mental illness. The paper says that 20% of travel incidents have been described as psychotic and according to WHO severe mental illness constitutes 1-3 main health crisis in air travel.

Stress, lack of sleep, crowded airports and culture shock are all known triggers for schizophrenia or psychosis. However, I've since made successful trips to Barcelona, Lanzarote and, more recently, (as seen in the issue!) caught a flight to Belfast!

Here are some tips that helped me:

MEDICATION, MEDICATION, MEDICATION, THAT'S WHAT YOU NEED!

It's crucial that medication is factored into travel to prevent relapse. As luggage can sometimes be lost you can take medication in hand luggage to keep it near at all times. For the stay, a pharmacy can sort out a scheduled pack of medication for each day. Don't forget to order any repeat prescriptions in advance to cover your time away.

PEOPLE HELP!

Whether it's taking a trusted friend to the airport for support, traveling with your love, or visiting a helpful neighbour pre-flight – the right people will and can reassure any travel nerves with humour or distracting anecdotes. If it wasn't for Paul's wonderful jokes or my neighbour Sonya's fine conversation and vegan pizza, I may not have made the flight to Belfast this year.

INSURE FOR THE BEST, INSURE FOR THE WORST

Mind have produced a detailed guide to travel insurance for mental health which is available freely on their website.

RELAX, JUST DO IT!

Try tested ways to relax during, before and after your journey: chamomile tea, lavender oils, deep breathing, and listening to soothing music on your headphones all help. When I flew to Barcelona from Liverpool there were even leather recliners with massagers built in to aid relaxation.

WHY EVEN BOTHER TO TRAVEL, YOU ASK?

A holiday abroad or at home has numerous benefits such as achieving goals, hopes and dreams. Learning about new cultures and switching primary identity from service user to tourist. With tenacious preparations, travel buddies, rest in-flights, plenty of water and avoiding alcohol, travel with severe mental illness is a very real possibility!

Cash-flow philosophy

By Stevie Shaw

'You need to buck your ideas up, sonny Jim,' shouted father. 'Money doesn't grow on trees, you know!' My father - always the practical realist.

Stephen didn't respond to the harsh reality check of his father. He was afraid to challenge his father's authority but, in his heart, he held his conviction that nature had real value whilst money did not. In his mind he said to himself; 'No father, but apples do and you can eat them. What use is money anyway, it's just pieces of metal and bits of paper.' Stephen knew well the words of Chief Seattle when he condemned the greed of the White Man; 'Only when the last tree is dead, only when the last buffalo killed and only when the last river is poisoned will you realise that you cannot eat money.

'You want to study philosophy?! What job will you get with that?' Stephen's father continued his barrage. Harold Leech, Stephen's college tutor chipped in too; 'Philosophy!? What will you do when you're shacked up with a woman and child?! How will you pay the bills?!'

'I'll be okay, I'll find something,' said Stephen in a weak voice, his head hung low. No one was convinced that this boy knew what was good for him.

Despondent from the meeting with his parents and teachers, and filled with doubt, Stephen took his leave to find some fresh air. It was late summer or early autumn. The leaves were going crispy. Big, crispy leaves everywhere. Stephen walked out past the old town walls, they were tall, maybe thirty feet high, built in medieval times and never used. Garden allotments filled a space between the town and the farmers' fields where herds of cows and goats, and flocks of sheep grazed behind stock fencing. Passing through the allotments with his mind depressed, Stephen noticed a solitary old man working his plot. Alone with his thoughts, Stephen wanted to mind his own business. To his utter surprise the old man called Stephen over, waving and calling. Stephen reluctantly complied. 'Come and sit down'. He offered Stephen his deck chair and said, 'Now, have some of this buttermilk. And tell me what the matter is.' Stephen told him about his worries for the future. 'How will I survive?' asked Stephen.

The old man opened his bible and showed Stephen a verse in Matthew; 'Therefore I tell you, do not worry about your life, what you will eat or drink; or about your body, what you will wear. Is not life more than food, and the body more than clothes? Look at the birds of the air; they do not sow or reap or store away in barns, and yet your heavenly Father feeds them. Are you not much more valuable than they? Even the pigeons get their daily bread, what to speak of the humans who are more dear to the Lord. The Lord provides for all of his creatures including the humans.

'Do not worry, do not fear, do not hesitate,' said the old man. 'Act to try and please the Lord and He will sustain you.'

This was music to my ears and just what I needed to hear. In his deck chair I had relaxed, assured to trust myself, and felt that God may have chalked my path. I gained a little confidence, and noticed my legs were stronger, less wobbly as I strode from the allotments. With the backing of the Christian man, I had the courage of my conviction, and would follow through with my desire to read philosophy. And to heaven with the consequences.

Stevie was a Hindu monk for 10 years living at an ashram on top of a hill in Scotland. He's been married seven years to his wife Geri who has schizo-affective disorder and, together, they have two beautiful daughters. He likes to speak about his experiences of being a monk, about religion, history and philosophy.

Balmoral chicken

By Erica Crompton

For a taste of Scotland, try this Balmoral chicken recipe complete with haggis, courtesy of Delicious Magazine. And for the best Balmoral chicken head to Kingsknowes Hotel in Galashiels, an imposing Scottish baronial mansion, built in 1869 for the local textile mill owner, Adam Lees Cochrane.

Ingredients:

- 4 free-range large skin-on chicken breasts
- 100g haggis
- 1 tsp freshly picked thyme leaves
- Knob of butter
- Splash of oil
- Serve with neeps and tatties (swede and potatoes)

For the whisky cream sauce

- 100ml chicken stock
- Splash whisky to taste
- 200ml of double cream

Heat the oven to 200°C/180°C fan/gas 6. Cut each chicken breast almost in half horizontally to form a pocket. Mash the haggis and thyme together in a small bowl with a fork (no need to season). Divide the mixture into four equal portions, then use to stuff the breasts. Use one or two cocktail sticks to secure the filling inside. Heat the butter and oil in the frying pan over a medium-high heat, add the chicken skin-side down and cook for about five minutes or until golden brown. Turn the chicken breasts over and brown the other sides for three minutes. Transfer the pan to the oven and roast for 15-18 minutes or until just cooked through (the juices will run clear when the chicken breast is pierced with a skewer in the thickest part). Remove the chicken and put on a plate to rest, loosely covered with foil to keep warm. Put the pan back on the hob, pour in the stock and use a wooden spoon to scrape up all the tasty, browned bits from the bottom of the pan. Stir in a splash of whisky and the cream, then season with salt and plenty of black pepper, adding a little more whisky to taste. Serve the chicken with neeps and tatties, steamed seasonal greens and a spoonful of whisky cream sauce.

Get yours ready-made and served piping hot – book a table at https://www.kingsknowes.co.uk/ or, for more information on dining in Scotland, check out VisitScotland.com.

Ardmore, the sea and me

By Graham Morgan

I must sound like a stamp collector! Nothing wrong with that, I say to myself, remembering a very distant childhood.

I collect sea glass - or sometimes I do. It is not good for my mental health like medication might be, or my CPN or doctor but it is good, like a walk in the woods, a good rest, a moment of bright laughter. I usually walk the shore on the Firth of Clyde in Argyll with Wendy, my partner. I would like to say soft sand and marram grass but really mud and pebbles. Still, it remains pretty idyllic.

Today, as I walked along, I could see seals on the rocks and the yellow of gorse flowers. In the summer, when there is a soft breeze and the butterflies and bees are everywhere, the waves ripple and the curlew's call; I like to sit among the pebbles to smell the sea. I listen to the wind and watch Wendy walking, peering intently at the ground, occasionally shouting with a weird glee when she finds a Bakelite bottle stopper or jewels of red, green, amber and blue sea smoothed glass.

I prefer to sit and swish my hands in the fine pebbles, vaguely watching ships on their way to I have no idea where. Idly picking up bits of sea glass, piling them in my lap to take home later. I like seeing the names of long-closed glass works on the jewellery. I like to find bits of crockery and imagine a family sitting down taking stew from the pot it once formed. Sometimes, as I walk, I come across the black heels of long-gone whisky bottles, almost like obsidian. I try to imagine what the bottle would have looked like but never quite succeed.

This - the breeze on my face; far off the sound of cars but here, bird song and gorse pods, cracking in the breeze. That smell of seaweed, the old wreck offshore, a murmur of conversation. I forget about the roar of my thoughts at night here. I forget about so much. I look up and smile at the person I now live with and walk back to the car hand in hand, thinking. even for people like us, life can be wonderful!

Graham Morgan is the author of Start, a memoir of love, life and schizophrenia. Available from all good bookshops and published by Fledgling Press.

Identity, disclosure and mental illness : how to tell people about your mental health at work

By Joe Tuesday

'Hi, my name is Joe and I have schizophrenia!'

Is that how you'd expect to start a conversation with someone you don't know? Would it shock you? Whether you are from within the mental health community or not it is quite a lot to comprehend on first meeting. It's like telling someone you're an alcoholic or recovering drug addict on first meeting.

Though fighting stigma is an excellent, just cause, is making mental illness the defining part of our identity really doing ourselves justice. As I disclosed at the beginning of the article, I have schizophrenia. I like to think I'm a pretty good person with lots of strengths. I have held jobs at four large corporate companies and hold a Bachelor's and master's in science from a good university but I am by no means exceptional. When you work with a mental illness the ownness is on the applicant to disclose their condition and this can mean all kinds of dealings with HR and occupational health. If not disclosing, the employer can sack you. With a disability, under equal opportunities, I may be entitled to an interview and can also ask for reasonable adjustments (for example flexibility with working hours) to help with my condition.

Communication with HR can be stressful. I remember one colleague I had said to me jokingly, that HR as well as standing for Human Resources stands for Human Remains, as that is all that is left of you by the time they've finished with you. It can feel a bit like that with so much scrutiny on your mental illness. Along with disclosure to your line manager comes disclosure to other colleagues, and this is where I would be very careful. I have disclosed to other colleagues in all my major roles and certainly, at one of my more recent companies, despite long loyal service, a wide variety of challenging job responsibilities over the years, I was not given a promotion. I feel this was due to disclosure of my mental illness to colleagues who subsequently blamed me for mistakes they made themselves and threw me under the bus when a discussion was being had.

Of course, this type of workplace bullying happens all the time, but I felt it all more acutely because of my association with mental illness. Going back to the start where I discussed social media, can you see how discussion of mental illness in your personal life, upfront on social media can creep into your professional life? Also how, although it is an important facet of my personality to understand, it should not be at the forefront of what I disclose to people!

Imagine if I put at the top of my CV, my name and brackets followed by 'comes with schizophrenia'. That would not be a good look, and I would probably never land a job again, despite the discrimination laws being in place in the UK!

It also helps to think of the reputation of some of these companies. I have worked for service companies in the past and some of their clients are notoriously difficult to work with. If word gets out to the client I have mental illness, I could be for the chop! Discrimination is not treated the same internationally and, after all, it is their product. Why would they want a schizophrenic working on it? It's a liability, right? So, my company would have to do the added job of selling it to them that I could perform, and, in my experience, they are completely unprepared, ill-equipped and even unwilling to do so. So, you see, disclosure in a work setting is not always simple, can play a role in your downfall and is really important to get right. I am a social media user and I see people who complain and say they struggle attaining employment and managing their jobs because of their mental illness. I'm not going to judge how it affects them, we are a broad church, some of us more afflicted than others. I just feel that fighting stigma as a one-man army and trying to hold down a career in what is very often a very scrutinised workplace is too much for most people and it is this mess with disclosure that is a big part of the problem.

This too can go for the dating world in our personal lives. I think it is the elephant in the room for a lot of people.

With love from Ireland : experiencing difficulty can positively impact you

By Caoimhe Clements

It was January 2021; the weather was cold and unkind, identical to my emotions. I was a university student in my final year, studying Photography with Video. With the pandemic creating a public health scare, the degree teaching of my final year took place completely online. No more in person teaching.

I enjoyed remote teaching it was comfortable but, at times, felt distant from my lecturers. It was the first time in my education career experiencing isolation from individuals on my course. The community and support of the university class was fully virtual which had an unpleasant atmosphere.

Stress began to pile up from remote teaching, covid restrictions and my freedom felt stripped from me. I was hit with a wave of emotional exhaustion, which soon led to my body taking seizures. Emotional exhaustion is experiencing high levels of stress, making a person physically worn out and drained.

This experience was powered with negativity and thoughts such as 'Why can't I handle my stress better?' and 'What did I do to deserve this?'. I soon realised the negative stress was controlling me, impacting my actions and emotions.

In order to build a healthier mindset, I needed a reason to hold myself accountable. Our mindsets are a reflection on how we think, feel and act. This was my motivation. I began to practice gratitude, focusing on reflective questions such as 'What is a positive in this situation?' and 'How can I make the outcome better?'. I traded in scrolling on my phone for books under the category of 'Personal Development'.

As time progressed, I became deeply interested in self-growth and seeking out new ways to challenge myself. I shared my story of emotional exhaustion and having seizures with people who were kind and loving. I realised my story was important and the idea of 'everyone has a story to tell' became embedded in my brain.

As a result, I made a podcast, launching in January 2022. I selected the name 'Optimistic Waves' – optimistic is to feel confident and hopeful about the future. The word waves refers to the act of riding the wave of emotions no matter what we experience. Each episode features a guest with an encouraging story to inspire listeners.

Being in a better place meant I returned to education in September 2022 to gain my master's degree in journalism. Journalism has a further power to tell stories that matter to people. This is the type of journalist I inspire to be.

About the writer:

Caoimhe Clements is 23-year-old Irish fine art photographer, writer and aspiring journalist. She graduated in July 2021, with a BA Hons Degree in Photography with Video, returning to university in September 2022 to gain her MA in Journalism. Caoimhe has an interest in psychology which influences the subjects and topics which she speaks about, including mental health, climate change and education.

An ode to Scotland : the place that will always feel like home

By Laura Menéndez

I vividly remember the day I stepped on a plane to change my life forever. After a year of university in Spain, I knew it wasn't for me. I accepted an offer to study in Scotland. And off I went. A big suitcase and a lot of hope accompanied me in my journey to my new life. I said goodbye to my parents for the first time in life.

My flight landed in Edinburgh late at night on a late August evening. The cold breeze hit me as I was leaving the aircraft, a cold breeze that from then on became a reflection of calm and stillness, of peace. I took the bus to the city centre, and Princess Street will always hold a special place in my heart. The big lights and the business of it welcomed me straight away.

It comes without saying to highlight the beauty of Scotland and its spirit. I fell in love with Edinburgh straight away. There's a certain magic surrounding the city, a sort of fairy-tale atmosphere that wraps you like a big hug, especially being a tourist who sees it for the first time.

My four years in university left me with a feeling of wanting more and, if there is one reason, I'd have to explain it is the people of Scotland. Rarely have I encountered in other places the warmth of heart of its people and its landscapes. The big hills and the way they change colour throughout the season is something I will always remember. Scotland can feel like a daunting place because of its weather, the grey winter, and the rain.

I have experienced Scotland in its prime summer sunshine, an ocean of green and yellow flowers, and as much as I love it there is always something remarkable about its gloomy rainy winter days. Again, like a fairy-tale.

Leaving a shop, whether it is after purchasing an on-the-go cup of coffee, mascara at Boots or having visited a local shop is something that very rarely fails to exist without a 'have a nice day' from whoever is on the other side of the counter.

It would be extremely complicated to describe Scotland in one single piece, but if there something that defines it, to me at least, is its warm heart. The warm heart of its people, who will, almost without a doubt, help you with a smile in their faces.

Bittersweet (a poem about relocating to Scotland from Spain)

By Laura Menéndez

In the busy morning of a train
I have found
Silence
-I was missing-

The quiet was daunting,
almost oppressing.
A monotonous fog
had taken over.

I had nowhere left to go.

In the silence and the quiet,
the stillness of one room,
in the perpetrating
emptiness
the darkness
was hard to avoid.

Dense particles of inconformism,
of tiredness,
loss of hope,
had invaded the corners of my house,
of my head
and my soul.

After navigating
the dark corners of the world,
of my world,

I arrived,
in peace,
and found stillness,
in having visited
the dark.

A glow of sunshine,
a rainbow in the rain.
A trip to the darkness,
a reflection on the sadness
that lives within me,
and may always stay.

A moment to appreciate,
that whatever happens,
brings me here,
to myself,
daily,
that even demons,
my demons,
deserve kindness,
patience.

I left the train,
hope
light
return to the surface.

The grey
though bittersweet,
left me
satisfied,
fulfilled,
content.

I had stared at the window
while navigating
the darkness
in the sky
in my soul.

I had come back
stronger,
brighter,
with a hunger for life,
nowhere to be found before.

For the life that shines
that fades
that always comes back around;
be brave,
be kind,
what's inside of you
is yours.

And even your sadness,
deserves moments
of light.

One hope, two kindred spirits

By Jason Rockyie Bissessur

The year I met Erica Crompton was the year I'll never forget. It was 2004, soon after finishing drama school when I got pied off by yet another friend who I thought was my 'best friend for life'. She thought I was sweet but weird, just not her cup of tea, and she loved her tea with no sugar. I found myself alone, no friends but with a big heart of gold. Suffering from anxiety at this point, I cried in my hands with my self-esteem at an all-time low. All I had left was hope.

I decided to join a foundation degree journalism course at the UAL London College of Communication, determined not to trip up on my shoelaces, searching for best friend 'number 236' (felt like that many). I saw Erica on my first day. I kept telling myself 'Don't be weird, don't be weird', trying not to look overly keen, and nervously strolled up to her. I said, 'Hello I'm Rockyie, nice to meet you' and plonked myself beside her. She had a lovely bright smile that could light up street-lamps in the dark and, when she shook my hand, something clicked. I didn't feel alone anymore, like two kindred spirits meeting at first light.

One conversation led to many, laugh after laugh. We'd make jokes and bond under the sun and stars. She was different to everybody I've met. She liked I was weird and vivaciously camp with jokes that went down like a lead balloon. I loved her sassy Erica-vibe: larger than life. She told me she had paranoid schizophrenia and believed she was Britain's most wanted criminal. 'I believe there's helicopters looking for me now', she said. I was all too intrigued. All these years I wanted a best friend like her, and I was all too happy to go with her on the run. 'Let's go on the run,' I said, to show her I was up for it. She laughed. I told her I had bad anxiety and got paranoid every time I smelt poo and my bottom would break into a sweat. Erica laughed so hard she almost cried. For the first time somebody was laughing with me, and not at me.

And 20 years later of liquid lunches, parties, catwalk shows, cat awards and laughs, my kindred spirit has remained till this day my best friend. Believe in hope.

CHAPTER THREE

HOPE FOR ALL DISABILITIES

Clatter of Jackdaw

By Eleanor Lees

Birdsong is something my blind friend has come to be able to identify - enjoying being able to tell me which songs are coming from which birds despite not being able to see them. She imagines them in her mind's eye and describes to me how she sees them.

The collective flight of birds is something I enjoy, being able to identify which birds are which from the way they move, and I wanted to share this with her in a poem so that she could also enjoy the beautiful swathe of a flock of birds moving together in her mind's eye.

Clatter of jackdaw

Close your eye
Watch with me in dark or
In brilliant white light
As I describe the
Clatter of jackdaw
Feverish flight of the pinkening night
Group-level consequence
Of not slowing for a corner too tight

In sublime Kinematics the initiators of self
Morphology
A story unfolds
The self-imposed spatial distancing for maximum velocity beholds
The scansion
Of ancestors

As starlings join crows, mobbed by the air
Thrifty clouds are fighting the pale blue descent
Dark under waxing moon crescent
My neck tingles tiny hairs

As a feather floats
To the foot of my foot
And I daren't look
Any more
At this private dance in the sky of skies
Now I close my beady eye

And I sense that you feel the feathers soft edge
More than I.

Belfast's Blue Badge Billy

By Erica Crompton

Opening a conversation with local residents is how you really get a feel for the charm and elegance of Belfast and a sense of how this UK city has emerged from conflict to become a safe, popular short-break city. Today it stands as one of the world's top tourist destinations thanks to the experience exhibition Titanic Belfast and Game of Thrones.

This month, I travelled for the first time to Belfast with my boyfriend Paul, who happens to use a wheelchair. Mindful of this, we found the best way to explore such a peaceful city is by a black cab. Specifically, a Blue Badge Tour Guide by Billy Scott, a fountain of local knowledge who, many times, broke out into song to relay local knowledge to us.

From the grand universities to the wall murals in the suburbs, this three-hour ride enabled Paul to see the city from the comfort of a black cab, his wheelchair folded with us in the back. The tour takes just under three hours and starts off in the university district, then meandering down residential streets where the upwardly mobile residents of Belfast live. We are able to stop off for a bathroom break and also to sign the Peace Wall, twenty minutes from the city centre.

The murals in the suburbs make for a fascinating but sobering historical tour. Billy tells us that the locals don't mind the taxi tours in their neighbourhood as it enables them to tell their story. As we travel back our hotel, where the journey started, Billy breaks into song again and it all ends on an uplifting note: 'Don't believe all I've just said!' He winks as we depart.

Billy Scott, Blue Badge Guide and Taxi Tour guide will collect you from your hotel for a special black taxi tour of the city (approx. three hours). For more information or to book Billy, visit https://touringaroundbelfast.com/

Quail birds at Edo restaurant

By Erica Crompton

'Is this the Quail or the egg?' It's only after sampling the vast array of local Belfast beers and whiskeys that I ask this, but the friendly staff take it in their stride: 'It's the bird,' offers the understanding waitress, all pristine black shirt, matching apron and compassionate smile.

EDŌ, pronounced 'aye-doh' is Latin for 'I eat' and this busy canteen-style restaurant offers tapas as well as more traditional main-meal and starter dining. Here you'll get a relaxed experience where you can enjoy the tastes from head chef and owner, Jonny Elliot, who's worked for everyone from Gordon Ramsay to Gary Rhodes. It's just three minutes' walk from the Belfast City Hall.

Paul and I visited this month and managed to master the doorway here fine with the wheelchair (there's a small step to get over). Sitting could have been more spaced, especially for accessing the bathroom, but the closeness of it all added to a cosy feel.

We tried six different dishes, three each, which was more than enough. A highlight was the black pudding and chorizo, chased down with an Espresso Martini. There are vegetarian options, too, if that suits you better. Personally speaking, I enjoyed the richness of the meats here. And the taste of the Quail made up for my embarrassing culinary question, too.

Visit Edo restaurant at Unit 2, 3, CAPITAL HOUSE, Upper Queen St, Belfast BT1 or call 028 9031 3054 to book. https://www.edorestaurant.co.uk

The Cringletie is the Scottish hotel that wins on accessibility

By Erica Crompton

As a white snow blankets the rolling hills that frame the River Tweed, we take a left from the scenic Edinburgh Road and over a private bridge to discover the Cringletie, a secluded baronial mansion. Snowflakes blanket the driveway as we pull in and we're helped with our luggage from the disabled parking to the lift-assisted entrance. A fire roars over tartan carpets to greet us and sets the tone for a warm and comfortable stay.

In all seasons, the Cringletie welcomes guests from all walks of life. Set in a 28-acre estate, amid the rolling hills of the Scottish Borders, just outside Peebles, and only around 20 miles from Edinburgh.

The venue is a popular choice for wheelchair users, being a fully accessible hotel that includes a range of facilities quite exceptional for a historic building. A small lift that shuttles us from the room to restaurant and an automatic wide door to the double bedroom, both being good examples.

Accessibility could be the Cringletie's trump card if it wasn't also so luxurious and accommodating for all. Designated parking is available close to the entrance with plenty of room for transport with additional space requirements, a wheelchair access ramp outside the house, an easy-to-operate chairlift to the ground floor, and a passenger lift to the first and second floors.

These facilities have won the **Catey Award for Accessibility**. 'We received the award some time ago, but very proud we can offer so much accessibility for our guests.' says Natalie Nisbet, Cringletie's Weddings and Events Manager, adding: 'In the house we have 13 bedrooms, nine are accessible and one of these is fully equipped specifically for wheelchair users with handrails, alarms, adjustable beds and chairs and a full wet room.'

Paul and I stayed this winter and enjoyed the cosy feel of the hotel as well as the hearty 'full Cringletie' Scottish breakfast with haggis and tatties. On those cold winter nights, we were spoilt with open fires in every room including the foyer, bar and restaurant. The devil is in every detail here from the roll-in shower, friendly staff and the adjustable armchairs where we reclined for our 'wee dram' of Scottish whiskey at the end of each night.

To book your stay, visit www.cringletie.com or, for more information on visiting Scotland, please visit www.visitscotland.com/holidays-breaks/accessible/

A special place

By Erica Crompton

'People that visit us here in Kailzie gardens all say it's such a special place,' says Steve, our accessibility guide for the afternoon tour of the gardens. There's a dedicated off-road wheelchair here that Paul uses, and Steve pushes today as we cast our eyes over walled gardens that punctuate the River Tweed, just a stone's throw north of the gardens.

Perhaps Kailzie is one for me though – the half of Paul and I with a mental illness. 'Forest bathing' has come over to the UK from Japan and is now quite the trend. If you're not familiar with this, it's simply spending time in tranquil nature and 'bathing' among trees and flowers, taking in the birdsong. An hour here left me feeling refreshed, and calm – it felt like a pleasant and far cry from my career days in London when the 10 lattes a day kept me awake but frazzled.

The River Tweed and the burn that flows through the garden provide an excellent habitat for birds such as the kingfisher, heron, oyster catcher, duck, wagtails and dippers. We spotted a heron here today, diligently and patiently waiting for his lunch on the river.

A highlight for me was the green arched bridge where Primula Pulverulenta had been planted, and two Cercidiphyllums (the Katsura Tree) on the bank provided wonderful colour which is said to be best in the autumn.

The off-road wheelchair enabled us to take the gardens in, in their entirety, with some steep slopes to content with (I was glad Steve was pushing the chair!). The tour ended at the site where an old and magnificent manor house once stood. Here is the most splendid view of the River Tweed and beyond and, according to Steve, it's the site most requested for ashes to be scattered. It's easy to see why: who wouldn't want to rest in these gardens so peaceful. Steve's feedback from guests is – it's a special place.

For more information visit www.kailziegardens.com or for more information on visiting Scotland, please visit www.visitscotland.com/holidays-breaks/accessible/

Gin Palace : DIY tipples overlooking the River Tweed

By Erica Crompton

It was back to school last month, with a seriously magical twist – Paul and I were visiting a wheelchair-friendly gin school where we learned to make our own gin, and try it, too! The school itself is set within the Hydro Hotel, in Peebles and is spacious and all lower-level. Set next to the hotel's spa, this school smells heavenly combined with the aromas of gin.

Our session kicks off with a large gin and tonic to welcome us, followed by an extensive tour around Hydro's very own distillery so we got to see exactly what happens at every step of the gin distilling process.

After inhaling a platter of amuse bouche, making our bottles of 70cl gin begins. The gin making equipment is a few steps up from the bar but there's a specially built lower-level gin-making table for Paul. The three-hour experience is designed to give adults a day experience while staying at the hotel.

Gin isn't easy to make, but with our friendly guide we're soon able to flavour the ethanol liquid (not to mention taste it – which is where the afternoon takes a turn!). From splash to sip, the gin school sits on what was once the original hotel swimming pool (a long, long, time ago). A lot has changed since then – these days we found 26 individual copper stills neatly lined in rows and glass jars brimming with botanicals – but the same water still flows down from the hills and into the Hydro as it did 140 years ago.

I was told that guide dogs and hearing dogs are always welcome at Peebles Hydro, too. Just don't mention the wheelchair push to the taxi – it was curvy to say the least!

To book your class visit www.1881distillery.com.

Fly me to the moon

By Erica Crompton

This winter, a trip to the ecclesiastical Durham Cathedral saw an art installation that is currently touring the UK. Luke Jerram's artwork, Museum of the Moon, illuminated the high vaulted ceiling and colossal carved pillars of the cathedral based in the north east.

At seven metres in diameter, the inflated moon installation is a fusion of 120dpi detailed NASA imagery of the lunar surface, moonlight, and surround sound composition created by BAFTA and Ivor Novello award winning composer, Dan Jones. Each centimetre of the internally lit spherical sculpture represents 5km of the moon's surface, at an approximate scale of 1:500,000.

The Reverend Canon Charlie Allen says, 'The moon looms large in the gifts of creation, the unsung backdrop of our daily lives. It reflects the sun bringing light to the darkness of night; its gravitational pull shapes the ebb and flow of the tides; its fullness defines the date of Easter. Here at Durham Cathedral, the moon's presence reminds us of our ancient foundation as a place of pilgrimage – a place in which awe abounds as we reflect with perspective on our own lives and rejoice in the wonder of being part of God's creation.'

Although the building of Durham Cathedral commenced in 1093, today it's been made accessible to wheelchair users, although the push to the top of the hill where the cathedral sits is tough on the lungs. As a person with experience of psychosis I also found the Museum of the Moon to be enormously relaxing to sit under – it felt meditative, but it was also nice that I could enjoy it with Paul in his wheelchair.

Accessibility of the Museum of the Moon artwork is intended, too, as Luke Jerram tells Hopezine: 'From my perspective, I try to make artwork that can be enjoyed by everyone.'

Find more information at www.durhamcathedral.co.uk or to find where the Museum of the Moon is on next visit https://my-moon.org/about/

A day in Durham

By Erica Crompton

Whether you're a nature lover, culture vulture or history buff, you'll find all this and more on a day out in Durham. Take in the historic streets of Durham City to the world-famous Durham Cathedral and Castle UNESCO World Heritage Site – an Instagram-worthy view dotted with small groups of students.

In the Durham Dales, explore themed galleries that showcase the stunning collections of fine and decorative arts at The Bowes Museum. At nearby Raby, discover one of England's finest medieval castles with its stunning 18th century Walled Garden. And in Bishop Auckland, enjoy the Deer Park, part of The Auckland Project, and follow in the footsteps of the Prince Bishops of Durham who created the park over 800 years ago.

If you prefer shopping to sightseeing, head to Dalton Park, the biggest outlet shopping centre in the north east. Or take in the charm of Durham City with its independent retailers. We recommend an accessible stay with accessible swimming pool at The Radisson Blu hotel, set along the River Wear. The only drawback is that the accessible rooms didn't have a walk-in shower which meant Paul had to wash in the sink. Not to worry: in all, we found Durham a quintessential English city peppered with historical and cultural charms.

A glowing green hotel

By Erica Crompton

Hope Street: Belfast's Holiday Inn lights up green in the evening which makes for an eerie entree. But we don't mind this at all as we enter, as it boasts both steps to the entrance and a step-free entrance for wheelchair users.

A bottle of Pinot Noir awaits with a handwritten note which is just as delicious. The devil's in the detail here – cushions are plump, the room's scent is sweet and we're overlooking a lovely mural of two national football players with the words: 'Welcome to our wee country!'

During a stay at the Holiday Inn here, you'll be minutes from the Grand Opera House and Ulster Hall. With four-stars, this hotel is also within close proximity of Linen Hall Library and St. Malachy's Church.

Make yourself at home in one of the hundreds of guestrooms, including the accessible guest room with roll-in shower, which Paul and I stayed in this month. Paul says he enjoyed the wet room, and the shower was easy to use with a built-in seat and large shower head.

We received complimentary wireless access, toiletries and a hair dryer as all guests do. There was also a fitness centre (that we didn't use!) and we ate breakfast every morning from a buffet – the lattes being exceptional though not included in the stay.

From eerie green beginnings to sorrowful endings (we were sad to say goodbye), this is one hotel that lights up more than just the entrance.

Book your stay at Holiday Inn in Hope Street, Belfast, at www.hibelfastcitycentre.co.uk

Accessible Stoke and North Staffordshire

By Caroline Butterwick

North Staffordshire has been my home for over a decade. I love exploring where I live, and I'm still discovering places to visit for a great day out. Being partially sighted and experiencing tiredness from medication I take for my mental health, accessibility is key when planning a trip. Luckily, there are lots of fantastic accessible attractions on my doorstep.

Whether curious about ceramics or a lover of the outdoors, here are a few ideas for accessible and enjoyable days out in Stoke-on-Trent and North Staffordshire:

- Trentham Estate - in the south of the city, the popular Trentham Estate has a range of activities to enjoy. The shopping village boasts dozens of independent and big brand stores and restaurants – I love the Portmeirion shop for swooning over pretty pottery.

Trentham Gardens is one of my go-to places in the area. The walking route around the mile long lake is well worth a go and is accessible to wheelchairs and buggies.

Some days, there's nothing better than a cappuccino and a fruit scone loaded with cream and jam. The Italian Garden Tearooms is the perfect place to enjoy an al fresco treat while watching the world go by.

Disabled visitors benefit from reduced entry fees and carer tickets. I have a Trentham Gardens annual pass and a free accompanying carer pass, which is great value and well worth it if you're planning to visit often. Also on the estate is Trentham Monkey Forest, where the 140 free-ranging Barbary macaques can literally cross the path in front of you – perfect for snapping some unique photos.

- Potteries Museum and Art Gallery - this is one of my favourite museums and where I take friends visiting the area. There are, of course, plenty of ceramics on display, with lots of info on the history of the pottery industry in the area. I also love the local history gallery, which recreates what shops and houses looked like in the past. There's good step-free access in the museum, with a hearing aid loop at reception. The staff are really friendly and helpful too.

- Alton Towers theme park - as a self-confessed theme park enthusiast, I love Alton Towers and am so glad we have this fantastic theme park nearby. From world beating rollercoasters to rides for the whole family, there is plenty to keep you busy.

Alton Towers has a Ride Access Pass for disabled guests who aren't able to queue in the standard line. Being disabled doesn't automatically entitle you to a pass, so be sure to check out their detailed accessibility guide beforehand to see if you are eligible and what evidence you'll need to bring.

The park is really spread out, and, as I struggle with tiredness, I tend to make a plan beforehand about what rides to visit. I also make the most of the cafes for regular coffee breaks so I'm ready for more rollercoasters.

A delightful day in York

By Erica Crompton

As one of the UK's biggest tourist destinations, Paul and I fiddled with chocolate buttons and ate like Fat Dan from Rate My Takeaway recently in York. For our stay, we drove 20 miles north east of the city centre to Sandburn Hall Hotel, which had the most sophisticated wet room we've yet to encounter on our travels for Hopezine. It was all gunmetal-grey tiles with a long mirror for wheelchair users and able bodies alike. See if you can spot Paul taking the photo! After a restful night's slumber, we had a full day ahead so a big breakfast buffet at Tykes restaurant was essential.

We took a ten-minute drive to Castle Howard for coffee and cake set in a beguiling stately home, all naked statues and historic artworks displayed with impeccable taste for interiors. Our next stop was York city centre for a City Cruise on an accessible boat. It's a lovely way to take in all the history and sites of York while bobbing along the canal, dotted with fisher people! One thing we learnt about on the cruise was York's world-famous chocolate industry and we explored this a little more in-depth at nearby York's Chocolate Story in King's Square. Here we had an entertaining tour of the site and got to add buttons and wafers to our own chocolate lolly sticks! We also watched with watering mouths as skilled chocolatiers gave a demonstration of chocolate making in action!

Our final stop in our tour of York is the Minster, one of the world's most magnificent cathedrals, and the largest gothic cathedral in Northern Europe. Since the 7th century, the Minster has been at the centre of Christianity in the north of England. Paul loves the accessibility of the place and we both enjoy the colossal stained-glass windows. Before leaving, we give thanks to all York has to offer by lighting a candle and saying a prayer.

Sent to a newly chic city

By Erica Crompton

With its recent reign of City of Culture, Coventry has had a revamp. Think flat streets: the silver lining to a rebuild after the World War II bombings. There's chic retro restaurants and the viral sensation that is Binley Mega Chippy, too. We went along to see what it was all about.

Our first stop was St. Marys Guildhall, a former prison to Mary Queen of Scots, and once a theatre for Shakespeare. Here in the Cathedral quarter of Coventry we found the ecclesiastical building has recently reopened after some work. Paul loved the accessibility that had been considered in the renovation and I loved the elephant icon that had been restored, too – you have to look closely around the building for little elephant signs!

Around the corner you'll find The Reel Store, part of a renovation of the former Telegraph Coventry newspaper site and The Telegraph Hotel's first permanent, immersive digital art gallery. We immersed ourselves in a digital exhibition by artist Refik Anadol that sees soothing projections of space imagery on the walls, floors and ceiling slowly moving around and covering all in the space.

After taking in the culture, we stopped for cocktails at the neighbouring Telegraph Hotel, another part of the former newspaper building's empire. Think luxury and fifties glamour straight out of the Mad Men TV series. We both enjoyed the Forme & Chase restaurant, bar and lounge here, especially the wide entrance complete with black marbled facade that harks back to the days of Fleet Street. To end our stay, we inhaled a refreshing cup of afternoon tea at Coombe Abbey Hotel set in a nearby 500 acres of parkland and formal gardens in the Warwickshire countryside. The site dates back to the 12th century and was surrendered to King Henry VIII during the dissolution of the monasteries and the future Queen Elizabeth I even lived there as a child – something to ponder over our cups of Earl Grey as the sun sets upon us.

CHAPTER FOUR

HOPE WITH A CRIMINAL RECORD

My Guiding Light

By Sobanan Narenthiran

In the veiled halls of existence, where shadows intertwine,
I walked, bound by karma, through the tapestry of time.
Within these walls of illusion, under the cosmic eye's gaze,
I found an ancient wisdom, a love that burns and blazes.

Unconditional love, the alchemist's stone, in my journey's night,
A beacon of mystic fire, guiding me with ancient light.
It whispered secrets of the universe, of cycles ever true,
A promise of enlightenment, in the celestial hue.

From my cell of flesh and bone, in this earthly plane,
This love was my compass, through loss and through gain.
Not defined by the material, nor by the chains of fear,
But by the capacity to transcend, to become the seer.

In the silence of the cosmos, under the watchful stars' flight,
I felt the cosmic embrace, transcendent and infinite, holding me tight.
It taught the dance of creation, strength in the ethereal,
Peace found in the cosmic order, in love's eternal spiral.

To those navigating the mysteries, on paths veiled and arcane,
This love awaits, timeless and profane.
It seeks not the mundane, but an open soul,
A guiding light for the seekers, making the fragmented whole.

This love knows no bounds, transcends time and space,
A beacon for the souls wandering in the cosmic chase.

It's the hand that lifts us to the heavens high,
A melody of the spheres, in the vast, unending sky.
So, to all who journey inward, seeking light in the dark expanse,
Remember, love is the mystic's dance.
It's the key to the mysteries, the flame in the cold,
A solace in the quest, the most sacred tale told.

Even in the labyrinth of being, where light seems lost in the maze,
Love finds a way to shine, to set the heart ablaze.
So hold to this beacon, let it guide your soul's flight,
Until you merge with the cosmos, in the dawn of eternal light.

Is time just an illusion?

By Sobanan Narenthiran

In the grand tapestry of existence, the concept of time has always fascinated and perplexed humanity. We measure it, chase it, and often feel we're running out of it. Yet, what if I were to tell you that time, as we understand it, is merely an illusion? This realisation was the cornerstone of my journey towards personal development, a voyage that transcended the conventional boundaries of hours and minutes, leading to a profound transformation within.

It all began on a seemingly ordinary day. The clock ticked in its usual rhythm, dictating the pace of life with its unyielding hands. Yet, amidst the monotony, a question lingered in my mind, 'Is time the architect of my destiny or just a construct of the human mind?'

This question propelled me into a quest for understanding, a journey that led me to ancient philosophies and the latest theories in physics, only to discover that time, as Einstein suggested, is indeed a relative concept, varying with perception and circumstance.

As I delved deeper into the nature of time, I stumbled upon the teachings of Eastern philosophies, which view time not as a linear progression but as a cyclical flow of moments. This perspective was a revelation, suggesting that the past, present, and future coexist, intertwining in the dance of existence. It dawned on me that, if time is fluid, then the power to shape my destiny lies not in the hands of an invisible clock but in the realm of my consciousness.

Embracing this concept, I began to see life through a different lens. The pressure to chase after future goals and mourn past losses diminished, making way for a profound appreciation of the present. I learned to live in the moment, understanding that each second is a gateway to eternity, an opportunity to enact change and foster growth. This shift in perception was liberating, freeing me from the shackles of chronological constraints and opening my eyes to the limitless potential that resides within the now.

With this newfound wisdom, personal development became a journey of being rather than becoming. I focused on cultivating mindfulness, embracing the art of meditation, and practising gratitude, recognising the beauty and lessons in every moment. The illusion of time had distorted my perception of progress, equating it with future achievements.

Yet, true growth manifested in the depth of my experiences, in the resilience built through challenges, and in the joy found in simple pleasures.

This journey taught me that time is not a foe to be battled but a concept to be transcended. By stepping out of the linear narrative and embracing the cyclical nature of existence, I discovered the true essence of personal development. It is not about reaching a destination or ticking off goals within a timeframe but about evolving with each moment, learning, and adapting in the eternal now.

In the end, the illusion of time revealed a timeless truth: that life is a series of present moments, each holding the key to enlightenment and transformation. As we navigate the river of existence, let us not be constrained by the illusion of time but be guided by the wisdom of being present, for it is in the here and now that we truly live, grow, and find our purpose.

An education

By Jen McPherson

University was my entire world. I thrived there both on and off my course. I edited the student newspaper, had a show on the student radio station and organised an international development summit. I loved my course – politics with international relations – and made friends from around the world. Then disaster struck. It started with depression but soon turned to mania. I became psychotic. I went from being an extroverted student to an introverted recluse. I could not get up in time for lectures nor read my books and write my essays. I could barely clean my teeth.

I left university in my final year and spent the next three years holed up in solitude in my flat getting more and more unwell. Meanwhile, the university – Warwick – kindly gave me a second, third, then fourth chance. Every year I was meant to be sitting my exams, I blew it. My full-time job was being mentally ill. Eventually, my chances ran out and I was told to withdraw from Warwick. I was distraught. I cried for days. It was as though someone had ripped out an organ.

What followed wasn't pretty. My psychosis reached a crisis point and I was arrested. I was eventually sectioned in hospital and diagnosed with bipolar disorder. I received treatment; medication and psychological therapy which helped me recover. The one thing on my mind throughout my recovery was my degree. It was too late to go back to Warwick so I thought I would have to start from scratch somewhere. Also, I would be in hospital for a while, which would surely prove to be a barrier to my education, or so I thought.

I called my department at Warwick and spoke to a member of their admin team. She suggested I do credit transfer at the Open University. She had thrown me a lifeline. I transferred my credit from Warwick to the Open University and I thus only had one year left to complete at the Open University. It gave me a reason to live again, it gave me hope. All those years wasted while mentally ill weren't wasted. I started studying again when I was sectioned as an inpatient in hospital. It gave me an escape and focus from the monotony of hospital life. It was life changing. The day I got my first-class honours degree, I cried, this time from happiness. The Open University had given me a second chance at my education. A second chance at life.

Abandon hope all ye who enter here

By Con Cord

Abandon hope all ye who enter here. Were those words actually attached to the police station, the court building, the prisons or probation offices I visited during the course of my criminal journey? No, they weren't. They actually refer to Dante's Inferno and an inscription above the gates of Hell.

Did I abandon all hope as I frequented those establishments? With hindsight......not quite, but very nearly.

It is often expressed that prison in itself shouldn't be a punishment. The confiscation of freedom is what is meant to fit the crime. That's okay if serving time is only a physical restraint. Anyone who has been imprisoned will know it's the psychological and emotional aspects that are the true casualties of being inside. I am a Lifer. I did 15 years before I was 'released'. Of course, it doesn't end there because then there are hostels, probation visits, the threat of recall. Do I resent the imprisonment or subsequent supervision? Hell no! I more than deserved to be banged up. What surprised ME was that, as a country and as a society, prisoners are allowed a second chance.

Each day - on numerous occasions - I ache because of the pain and misery I caused. But each day, too, I am eternally grateful that people I hardly knew, people I seldom met, thought they could make a judgement call and conclude I had served my time and made me a 'free man'. Free in name only? No. Free to choose the life I want to live........ within the restraints of being an ex-offender. Am I bitter, resentful, angry? No, no, no!!

Upon release I left my old life behind. I had a clean slate, a blank canvas. I had gained knowledge from prison education courses, books, conversations with staff, fellow inmates and prison visitors. The world had new meaning. Living had a greater focus, a more profound sense of purpose. Over time and with much self-reflection, I discovered my own failings; I now play to my strengths. Prison life gave me an insight that not everyone possesses.

If you are an ex-offender - YOU have it too. It's not a superpower, but YOU have the ability to wield it and to allow it to overcome good over evil. That is YOUR power. Because of your time served you know right from wrong. You are not naive. Unlike a lot of the general public, YOU know where the pitfalls are. You know your weaknesses. You know the consequences if you go off-piste.

Believe it or not.... there are a great many people out there who just sleepwalk into danger. You, however, have your eyes wide open. Your senses are finely attuned to assess risks. You can navigate a safe course through a hazardous path. That is a tremendous skill. It is priceless. And the beauty of it is that it is locked away in your subconscious.

As ex-offenders are we disadvantaged? In some respects, yes. Does society, in general, view us with contempt? Undoubtedly. Unfortunately, society's perception of you is not their problem. Your guilt, oppression, remorse, or a whole range of other emotions that you carry are yours alone. You cannot shed them... and neither should you. Your experiences of life make you into the person you are today.

I guarantee you are your own worst critic. You agonise day and night about what you've done. But you know what? You can't undo the past. Embrace your offences, no matter how hurtful or shameful they may be. Don't let them define you but accept they have shaped you and sent you on a different course in life. I sometimes wish I could erase my past and start again. Sadly, that is not an option. I detest the person I once was. It's almost as if I have a toxic conjoined twin attached to my very being and I cannot remove the apparition without destroying my whole self in the process. Therefore, my solution to the enigma is this: don't jettison the baggage that threatens to weigh you down with its overpowering burden. Instead, scoop it up. Cradle it. Carry it as if it's a precious cargo; a piece of your sentient being. Why? Because it is an integral part of who you are. It will accompany you on your entire journey until you die. It is not your enemy. It is your closest, most intimate confidante. Allow it to guide you. Nurture you. Embolden you.

Ultimately, love the person you are today. You cannot alter your past wrongdoings. But you survived a traumatic experience and, as a survivor, it is never too late to change, to learn, to prosper. You have an incredible attribute - put it to good use and make your life meaningful, worthwhile and a celebration of why we are allowed to savour the joys of living. Let the embodiment of your prison life structure your daily civilian life in a positive way to ensure the remainder of your time on this wonderful planet is a blessing and not a curse.

Addiction ditty

by David Bayliff

Addiction is cruel, that's the main rule.
Abstaining from the vein, is the ultimate aim.
Whether inhaled, ingested or intravenous injected.
Drugs don't discriminate who are infected.

Loneliness lies and broken family ties.
No trees of green, just dark cloudy skies.
Whatever ya poison, it's basically the same.
Nobody lives long in this perilous game.
So, a trip to the quack, to get off the smack.
No cannabis, alcohol, vallies or crack.
Life finally feels better without all this junk.

I'm progressing, not stressing or perfecting to be a monk.
So off to inspire coz I'm ready to retire.
Hopefully get tools, set goals, gain desire.
Discover, recover, turn over a new leaf.
At last, I've no need for a criminal brief.
It's time to grow up, I'm no Peter Pan.
Time to build a recovery plan.
Motivation, dedication and desire to change.
Nothings impossible, it's all within range

Apple tree philosophy

by Just Ben

Do we live in a fallen world? What is the evil at work? Did God intend it this way?

This is something I have contemplated and prayed about. As with all things of God, I have found a lot of paradox when seeking an answer. I believe that I have been led to an understanding by God's trees and forests. I love how all creation shares the wisdom of God. As the Proverb says: 'Wisdom cries aloud in the street, in the markets she raises her voice; at the head of the noisy streets, she cries out; at the entrance of the city gates she speaks.'

Yes, we are fallen and that is the problem but it is not really a problem at all. Let me share as briefly as I can what I have discovered. A fruit finds itself high up in the branches of its parent tree. It enjoys a direct connection to its parent, it is fed, it grows, it is protected and it enjoys the light of the sun. One day, the fruit falls. It falls way down to the earth. It is disconnected from its parent, deep in the shadows of the forest away from the light of the sun, seemingly abandoned. The fruit begins to decay. It finds itself surrounded by other decaying fruits. Some of the fallen fruits are eaten up by the beasts of the forest. For the fruits this is suffering, even hell like. Eventually the fruit decays completely.

It now realises that it was not a fruit at all but is actually a seed. The seed sinks into the earth, into darkness.

The seed has no idea what is happening to it. This experience appears punishing, even cruel, to the seed. After a long time in darkness, the seed breaks open. It still does not understand what is happening but it reaches upwards towards the surface and towards the light.

Eventually with perseverance, the seed breaks through into the light and begins to grow upward. The seed now sees that it is not a seed at all but a small plant. The small plant continues to grow until it becomes a sapling, a baby tree. As it grows and gains height, it is able to look down to the forest floor. There it sees freshly fallen fruits, decaying fruits, and tiny plants emerging from the darkness. It begins to see that the decaying fruits are actually enriching the soil, enabling the growth of the forest and all in it.

The sapling sees that even the poop of the beasts who eat some of the fallen fruits enrich the soil and that, for some seeds, passage through the gut of a beast is necessary for that type of seed to germinate and grow. The sapling, through its roots, connects again to its parent. Through its branches and leaves it connects again with the light of the sun. The sapling begins to see the perfection of all things. The fruit was never a real fruit, never really a seed, never really a sapling, it is not even really a tree. It is a child of the forest. Throughout its development, no matter how it may have seemed or appeared to the fruit or seed, it was always a part of the forest, never disconnected. It lived, moved and had its very being in the forest. All things were always working together for the good and growth of the children of the forest. Yes, the fruit enjoyed a place in paradise while it hung in its parent's branches. But if it was ever to become all it could be, it had to fall to the earth. The fall was the greatest blessing ever bestowed on the fruit.

Prison is hope

by Samsara

Prison was the beginning,
the lowest of the lows,
I remember telling my mum,
the only thing worse was death,

It's difficult to think of a punishment so pointless,
Yet, an experience that makes your life a mess,
My first day in prison was hard, I felt so deeply lost,
When you think about crime, you never think of the cost,
The tears from your loved ones, the pain to yourself,

It's like for a moment, your life is on a shelf,
My life was on pause, for the sentence there was no remorse,
I just wanted to get back on the right course,
What was right? What was wrong? Why did the judge decide to give me so long?

I wasn't a bad person, I was a lost kid,
Weed doesn't kill, it was the only thing I allegedly did,
I remember what my teacher said, Prison was the best worse thing,
I learnt about the sorrow, the loss of freedom is a sting,
Prisons could be a place of hope, but instead they are despair,
Most of the people, they wouldn't be there if life was fair,
Hurt people, hurt people, lost people chase fear,
Imagine, if you didn't know what to hold dear?

I wish that everyone cared about those in our prison walls,
Society would have chance, to save so many lost souls,
People are people, neither good nor bad,
In prison, we just guarantee that we'll make people sad,

Everyone is someone's child, sometimes they cause pain,
Only if we are willing to teach them, will they learn to refrain,
Prison made me a teacher, a monk and gave me my fate,
It was the School of Life, at least I had a release date,
13 Over time, I learnt to find meaning in my sentence length,
To feel wronged and to let go, this requires a deep strength,

If you're still inside, I beg you to engage,
Just learn to let go, there's no use in the rage,
You are a human, infinite potential locked in flesh,
Learn to live in a way, to be healthy and fresh,

Your life has value and you can achieve anything,
Your mind must be pure, you must begin dancing,
Each person in prison, can become a beacon of hope,
The first step is to get off the dope,

Then learn every day, read everything, become a master,
Once you are released, you will realise why, the real mission is to avoid disaster.

Yogic gardening

by Brian Bhakti McCulloch

My childhood wasn't too bad, apart from my father's drinking. My parents loved me and I loved them. But due to pressures of life, my father drank a lot and my mother ended up joining him drinking at the weekends.

By the time I was 17, I couldn't stay in the house at the weekend so I spent the weekends drinking in friend's houses. It wasn't long before I got into trouble with the law. I got three months detention for smashing some things up in a pub. The detention centre was tough: no talking to other inmates, army glasshouse training, marching, working hard and running a mile at six in the morning. The government closed it just after I left because of suicides.

When I got out, I hitched around the UK and ended up in London. I got a job in Debenhams in the cafeteria. While working there, some friends and I went out drinking and one friend smashed an off-licence glass door and stole some booze. The cops arrived and, after a short scuffle with them, I was arrested and given six months in jail.

When I was released, I was arrested at the gate of the prison in England and flown to Scotland. I arrived in Scotland and was sent to jail to await trial. I spent one month in jail then was found not guilty. So, I went back to London and was living in squats and hanging out in the West End.

There's a Krishna temple in Soho there, so a lot of young people used to go there and sing and dance and get a big feast of delicious vegetarian food. This was my life saver! I should have stayed in the Krishna temple because, before long, I was back in Brixton prison for a smash and grab and assault. After ten weeks in Brixton, I was found not guilty and released. After that, both my parents died. They were both only 52 years old each and I was heartbroken.

I had drifted away from friends. I ended up homeless, because I used to go and stay with my parents when I got fed up getting into trouble. I was trying to stay out of trouble but, due to bad company, I ended up in trouble again. I ended up banged up abroad! Luckily, the jail in Switzerland wasn't too bad, although due to bad behaviour I ended up in solitary confinement. I was in a real bad way in jail in Switzerland. I seemed to have lost all sanity and wasn't using my intelligence. I felt ghostly haunted, somehow or another I started chanting some mantras I'd learned at the West End Krishna temple. It seemed Krishna (a name for God) had listened to my calls for help: my lawyer came to visit me just after I'd been chanting and told me he could get me out.

I was flown back to London and went to stay in a squat where there was heroin and was offered some money to beat someone up for robbing someone who lived in the squat. I declined the offer and travelled back to Scotland, where I got a job in a garden centre. Next, I went to stay at the Krishna temple at the weekend and worked on the land. I moved into the Krishna temple and then got married and moved into a house on the Krishna Eco Farm property.

I haven't been in trouble with the law for 25 years now. I'm grateful to my family and friends who have shown me love over the years. I'm also thankful to the government for giving me the opportunity to train as a gardener for four years at a horticultural therapy project run by the Scottish association for mental health. I'm thankful to the devotees of the Krishna movement who have given me the chance to pay my debt back to society. I'm thankful to God (Krishna!) for giving me a second chance. I now spend my time teaching people 'bhakti yoga' in the garden at the Krishna Eco Farm. Bhakti yoga is the yoga of love: I teach people how to grow flowers fruit and veg with love. I've recently written my first book called Gardening the Bhakti Yoga Way. If anyone would like to get in contact with me, my email is in the book. I'm more than happy to help, no matter what the problem is. Hare Krishna!

Gardening the Bhakti yoga way: A gardening therapy book by Brian Bhakti McCulloch is available from Amazon.co.uk

How can you re-emerge from prison and successfully reintegrate into the community?

by Samsara

When I left prison, I was anxious, stressed and worried - it wasn't going to be easy. The stigma of being an ex-offender coupled with being young scared me: how would I get a job? How would I tell people where I'd been for the last year? How would I deal with all the people who had seen my article in the local newspaper?

These questions moved around my mind, leaving me in a daze. I want to provide a step-by-step guide to becoming successful after leaving prison, it will vary depending upon your own situation but I want to be as general as possible to ensure as many people can gain value from this as possible.

1. Don't be ashamed of your lived experience. It's easy to get caught up in what other people think, instead reframe this into what you think about yourself. If you've made progress in your personal development through taking responsibility for your life and making changes then speak about how your experience enabled you to achieve this. Your lived experience is just an experience, it doesn't define who you are unless you let it.

2. Educate yourself through freely available resources such as Youtube, social media, free courses, training through probation or other providers. It's pivotal that you engage with your own self-development: the only

way to overcome the barriers of a criminal record is to defy expectations. Knowledge is power. If you recite this mantra to yourself, you can motivate yourself to learn absolutely anything.

3. Your thoughts become your words, your words become your actions and your actions become your habits. It's a simple process in which you have full control - if you consume positive and productive content, you will produce thoughts that reflect this. It's key to remember that the music, films, media and people you immerse yourself in will determine how you think and how you perceive the world. Therefore, remain mindful and build good habits. If you want to know how your life will look five years from now, just take a look at your daily habits.

4. Focus on the present moment. It's easy to get wrapped up in the past and anxious about the future - instead, use simple exercises like meditation and journaling to anchor yourself to the present. The infinite present moment is all we ever have, don't lose precious time to the illusions of the past and the future.

5. Think about how you can serve the world. A key way to live that I've found useful since my release is to constantly think about how I can be of service to others. Whether it's as simple as picking up a piece of litter or offering someone support - learning to live in service can help us to forget our own troubles and give. To conclude, our journeys when we are released from prison can vary greatly. I believe that being a person who has been to prison is a strength, it gives you a unique insight into our society. Use that voice, to help create a system that's more compassionate and loving to those who need it.

ABOUT THE AUTHOR

Erica Crompton is author of The Mind Surfer, and co-author of The Beginner's Guide to Sanity with Professor Stephen Lawrie. She holds a master's degree in creative writing and undergraduate degrees in fine art and journalism. Erica lives with schizo-affective disorder and works part-time around this. She's written about living with a mental illness for The Los Angeles Times, The New York Times, The Mail on Sunday and The Guardian but she's also an avid fashion writer. In this capacity, she's penned pieces for The Daily Telegraph, Nylon, Vice, Vogue.co.uk and, more recently, has written regularly for The Daily Star in the UK. Currently she runs a small magazine called Hopezine with her boyfriend, a wheelchair user, and it covers inspiring stories of people overcoming adversity with disabilities, suicidal thoughts and prison sentences. She lives in an accessible bungalow in Staffordshire, with her partner Paul and two adopted cats called Caspar and Winter.

Printed in Great Britain
by Amazon